# ADRENAL FATIGUE

# CARMA
books

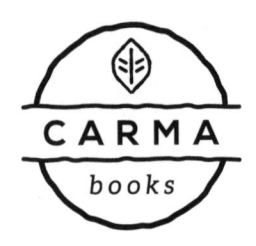

*'A conscious approach to health & wellness'*

**carmabooks.com**

*You are invited to to join our **Free Book Club** mailing list. Sign up via our website to receive **special offers** and **free for a limited time** Health & Wellness eBooks!*

# ADRENAL FATIGUE

## CURE IT
## *Naturally*

A FRESH APPROACH

*Reset Your Metabolism, Regain Energy & Balance Your Hormones through Diet, Lifestyle & Nutrition*

**PLUS BONUS RECIPES**

Carmen Reeves

*Copyright © 2015 Carma Books*

All rights reserved. No part of this publication may be reproduced, distributed, or transmitted in any form or by any means, including photocopying, recording, or other electronic or mechanical methods, without the prior written permission of the publisher.

*Disclaimer*

This book provides general information and extensive research regarding health and related subjects. The information provided in this book, and in any linked materials is for informational purposes only, and is not intended to be construed as medical advice. Speak with your physician or other healthcare professional before taking any nutritional or herbal supplements. There are no 'typical' results from the information provided - as individuals differ, the results will differ. Before considering any guidance from this book, please ensure you do not have any underlying health conditions which may interfere with the suggested healing methods. If the reader or any other person has a medical concern or pre-existing condition, he or she should consult with an appropriately licensed physician or healthcare professional. Never disregard professional medical advice or delay in seeking it because of something you have read in this book or in any linked materials. The reader assumes the risk and full responsibility for all actions, and the author or publisher will not be held liable for any loss or damage that may result from the information presented in this publication.

*Carma Books*
carmabooks.com

hello@carmabooks.com

# CONTENTS

**INTRODUCTION** ............................................................. 8

### CHAPTER 1
***About Adrenal Glands & Hormone Production*** ................. 12

*Cortisol Hormone* ........................................................ 14

### CHAPTER 2
***What is Adrenal Fatigue?*** ....................................... 16

*What Causes Adrenal Fatigue?* ................................... 17
*Four Levels of Adrenal Fatigue* .................................. 19

### CHAPTER 3
***Overlooked, Misdiagnosed, Misunderstood*** 22

*Adrenal Insufficiency Versus Adrenal Fatigue* .......... 22
*History of Adrenal Fatigue* ........................................ 23
*Illness-Wellness Continuum* ...................................... 24
*Subclinical Versus Clinical* ........................................ 26
*Large Patient Pool* .................................................... 27
*Medical Evolution* ..................................................... 28

### CHAPTER 4
***Adrenal Fatigue. Do You Have It?*** ................... 29

*Signs and Symptoms of Adrenal Fatigue* .................. 29

*Testing (or Lack There of)* ............................................. 33
*Self Diagnosing* ............................................................. 39

## CHAPTER 5

***Curing Adrenal Fatigue Naturally:***
***Diet, Vitamins & Supplements*** ........................ 42

*Diet* ................................................................................ 43
*Supplements and Herbal Support* ............................. 58

## CHAPTER 6

***Curing Adrenal Fatigue Naturally:***
***Sleep, Rest & Exercise*** ........................................ 66

*Sleep and Sleep Hygiene* .............................................. 66
*Rest, Relax and Reduce Stress* .................................... 68
*Exercise* ......................................................................... 71

## CHAPTER 7

***The Road to Recovery*** ........................................... 74

*Recovery Process* .......................................................... 74
*Willingness to Change* .................................................. 76
*Feeling Like Yourself Again* ......................................... 77

## CHAPTER 8
***Bonus Adrenal Support Recipes*** ...................... 79

A WORD FROM THE PUBLISHER .......................... 94

# INTRODUCTION

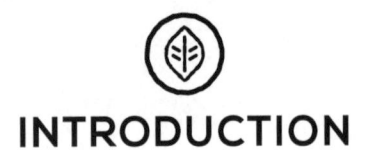

We live in a fast paced world of deadlines, competition, social and economic pressures, busy schedules and stress. Many of us often find our minds and bodies 'crashing'. *We. Just. Can't. Take. One. More. Step.* We also often view this "forced" slow-down period as an inconvenience, albeit a painful one, a distraction that gets in the way of getting things done. And just as soon as we can, we get up, and start doing it all, all over again, until the next crash. Sound familiar?

Have you ever wondered if this might be your body sending you a message? The fact that you've decided to read this book suggests the answer is yes. And I agree. Whether you are overloaded at work, dealing with stress or grief, enduring social pressures or recovering from an illness, over time your body can suffer long-term consequences with a slew of symptoms that emerge when we least expect it, or when it is least convenient.

If you are exhausted, stressed, incapable of sustaining the energy needed for your regular day-to-day activities; if you notice unexplained weight gain, it is possible that your adrenal glands are functioning at a lower than normal level. Adrenal Fatigue Syndrome leaves you feeling worn out and unable to function as efficiently as you once did. Adrenal Fatigue can devastate and disrupt your life.

Adrenal Fatigue Syndrome, a silent modern-day condition, is often overlooked or misdiagnosed despite being common and prevalent in today's society. For those of you who have taken myriad physical complaints to your medical doctors, only to be told "there's nothing wrong", or "it's in your head", and who have gone on to do our own research and take your own action to improve health (because you *KNOW* there is something wrong) - Adrenal Fatigue is indeed real, with real and negative health consequences on quality of life.

I know, because I've been there. I had what seemed to be a successful career: a high profile company, a decent income and high responsibility. But, as time passed, I realized how stressful my work life had become. Sleepless nights, tight deadlines, and workplace tension were the norm. My life had become completely unbalanced. I felt frazzled, worn out and constantly anxious. What seemed to be a great job from the exterior (to friends and family) became the thing that made my stomach twist and turn just thinking about it. Only I knew how stressful it really was, and how daunting it was to walk into work each morning in such a competitive environment.

My healing journey has been long and arduous. I didn't find the full support I needed from the medical community, so I took matters into my own hands and researched and experimented with various methods, as somewhat of a self-made guinea pig. In my desperate attempt to lose weight and feel well again, I tried everything; from restrictive diets through to painstaking juice fasts. I continued to read countless books and scientific studies, researched diet, herbal supplements, stress relief and how to exercise. Finally, I have found the methods that worked for me, and I have managed to successfully turn my health around.

My aim in writing this book is to save you the hard work and trouble I went through. With your long-term health in mind, I want to help you address the **cause** and help you avoid quick-fix approaches that will merely mask your symptoms, which as I discovered, can often exacerbate the condition and make it worse.

This self-help book will serve as a comprehensive guide to understanding Adrenal Fatigue, its causes, and recognizing its signs and symptoms. It will also offer a range of proven remedies for recovery. Through the power of lifestyle, diet and nutrition, you will learn to heal Adrenal Fatigue **naturally**, to reset your metabolism, lose weight and gain back your energy and happiness. I will show you how to do this without drugs, medications, or other stimulants that are temporary, short-term fixes that can actually prolong or worsen the condition.

This book explains in detail how to diagnose the syndrome, improve sleep patterns, how to manage stress, and how to nourish your body with the right diet and herbal nutrition, including some bonus recipes to help you kick-start your journey.

I understand your frustration and what it's like to feel 'crazy' due to being misdiagnosed and misunderstood after several visits to various doctors and practitioners. Throughout my journey of self-healing, I have documented the research and methods that have helped me on my road to recovery, and I share this information with the optimism that you can combat your Adrenal Fatigue too. Get ready to be empowered, and to embark on your journey to an energized and happy life!

# CHAPTER 1

## About Adrenal Glands & Hormone Production

Before we get to the good stuff that will help you heal Adrenal Fatigue naturally, it's important to first understand what the adrenal glands are, how they work, and what role they play in a healthy-functioning body. It's a little intensive, but bear with me. This will help you better understand why and how some of the treatments I recommend work.

Adrenal glands are a key component of what's called the HPA Axis: the hypothalamus, pituitary, and the adrenal glands. These three glands work together in a feedback loop to manage and regulate metabolism and energy levels, libido, immune system, mood and stress response.

### *Hypothalamus*
The hypothalamus, located deep in the forebrain, produces and secretes the hormone "corticotrophin-releasing factor", or CRF, in response to stress. The more stress, the more CRF is generated by the hypothalamus.

### *Pituitary*
The pituitary sits below the hypothalamus. As the hypothalamus secretes CRF, it stimulates the pituitary to release adrenocorticotropic hormone (ACTH), which travels to the adrenals and kidneys.

## Adrenals

The adrenals are walnut-sized glands located just above each of the kidneys and they play a big role in your overall wellbeing. (The root of the word "adrenal" comes from the Latin "ad", or near, and "renes", which is kidney.) They respond to the messages from the pituitary by producing hormones or chemicals that regulate the metabolism, inflammation and immune response.

Each adrenal gland is comprised of two distinct parts, with distinct functions.

## Adrenal Cortex

This is the outer layer, or shell, of the gland. Its job is to produce hormones that affect metabolism and other chemicals in the blood.

## Cortisol

Cortisol is one of the stars of the glucocorticoid family. Cortisol is famous for triggering our physical stress response to depression, anxiety, and excess exercise, lack of sleep or trauma. Cortisol stimulates norepinephrine, sometimes called noradrenaline, to put the body into "fight or flight" mode. I will address more about cortisol in a moment.

## Aldosterone

Aldosterone regulates potassium and sodium levels, and helps to maintain blood pressure and blood volume.

## Androgenic Steroids (Androgen Hormones)

The androgenic hormones, including DHEA (dehydroepiandrosterone), produced in the adrenal cortex are converted into female hormones (estrogen) or male hormones (androgens and testosterone), and they are also produced elsewhere in the body in larger quantities.

### *Adrenal Medulla*
This inner core of the adrenal gland is responsible for producing the hormones that help us cope with emotional and physical stress.

### *Epinephrine (Adrenaline)*
Epinephrine facilitates blood flow to the muscles and the brain, helps convert glycogen to glucose in the liver, and increases both the heart rate and the force of heart contractions.

### *Norepinephrine (Noradrenaline)*
This is the hormone that results in vasoconstriction, the squeezing of the blood vessels, which helps maintain or increase blood pressure when in acute stress.

## Cortisol Hormone

Cortisol, the stress hormone, is the most important hormone in the body's response to stress. Cortisol helps keep the body in balance, called homeostasis, by moderating or regulating activation of the central nervous system, anti-inflammatory and immune responses, glucose or blood sugar levels, blood vessel and heart contractions and tone, and as referenced earlier, the metabolism of fat, protein and carbohydrates.

If it is important for the adrenals to produce more cortisol in response to stress, it is equally important for body functions and cortisol levels to fluctuate and return to a normal state after the stressful event has passed. This is partly what gets mess up with Adrenal Fatigue Syndrome.

In our high-stress culture, often the circumstances of our lives don't generate this "return to normal" signal on that HPA axis feedback loop.

When the adrenals become overworked, producing too much cortisol, they start to exhibit signs of wear and tear, unable to keep up with the demand. When this happens, cortisol levels drop and the body and brain are no longer able to effectively respond to stressful or high-pressure situations.

### *Connection to the Thyroid*
The thyroid and cortisol hormones have a very close relationship. They work in tandem to make sure the body has enough energy. Hypothyroidism, where the thyroid doesn't produce enough thyroid hormone, is a very common condition. Prescription drugs may help restore the thyroid balance in many patients, but not in all. In patients who do not respond to this supply of bio-identical or desiccated thyroid, the symptoms of brain fog, anxiety, stress and low energy often persist. The missing link is often Adrenal Fatigue.

# CHAPTER 2

## What is Adrenal Fatigue?

Based on what you've read so far, you'll know that it's a stress condition. Adrenal Fatigue is an umbrella term for a group of symptoms that are caused by the adrenal glands no longer working at their optimum, and as a result, they fail to produce sufficient amounts of critical hormones needed by the body. When the adrenals stop performing properly, all parts of the body are affected.

In healthy, low-stress people, the feedback loop of the HPA axis works harmoniously. But, when there is chronic overproduction of cortisol and norepinephrine, the system becomes desensitized, or immune, to the negative messages to "calm down". This is what eventually leads to chronic stress on all three glands and often results in a number of fatigue conditions.

The overwhelming major symptom of Adrenal Fatigue is fatigue, especially with difficulty waking up in the morning. You may also experience weight gain or difficulty losing weight, sudden or abrupt weight loss, cravings for sweet or salty foods, hair loss, low blood pressure, recurrent infections and slow healing.

We'll get into more detail about the signs and symptoms of Adrenal Fatigue in Chapter 4.

## What Causes Adrenal Fatigue?

Western society is increasingly fast-paced, and it is simply more difficult than it was, even 50 years ago, to take a break and rest. Not just physically, but emotionally and mentally. Things like technology, where our devices follow many of us to bed, career pressures, relationship and family issues, can all add up to generate a constant stream of stress. At a certain point many of us stop being able to adequately respond when heightened or serious stress events occur, and sometimes this leads to an inability to cope or function with the stresses of day-to-day living.

Boiled down to basics, stress causes Adrenal Fatigue. Your adrenal glands simply become less and less able to cope with the hormone-production demands stress is placing on them.

What causes Adrenal Fatigue in one person may be quite different from the cause in another. Pinpointing the exact cause can be difficult. The signs and symptoms develop slowly, sometimes over a decade or more. It is not uncommon for someone to suffer Adrenal Fatigue Syndrome and never really know exactly what the trigger was. There are a number of causes that can be grouped into six major categories, in no particular order:

### *#1: Trauma*
A single, physically traumatic event can lead to Adrenal Fatigue, which sometimes manifests years later. Car accidents, major surgery, serious sports injuries or other

events all fall into this category.

### #2: *Chronic Disease*
Coping with chronic illness or disease places above-normal demands on your adrenal glands. Fibromyalgia, chronic pain, Lyme disease, asthma, diabetes or arthritis may all be factors.

### #3: *Not Enough Sleep*
Most recent surveys suggest Americans are getting an average of just over 6 hours of sleep per night. That's down from an average of 8 hours of sleep every night 50 to 100 years ago, and short of the 8 – 9 hours of rest the experts suggest we need before we are at risk of developing sleep disorders and other related illnesses.

### #4: *Emotional Stress*
Different from the stress caused by physical trauma, emotional stress may feel manageable in the short term. However, extended periods under emotional stress can cause, or at least contribute to, Adrenal Fatigue. Whether it's a bad boss at work, an unhappy relationship, having a sick child, moving, or the death of a family member, emotional stress can become chronic if the underlying cause isn't dealt with.

### #5: *Poor Diet, Crash Dieting & Addictions*
You've heard the saying 'you are what you eat'. Unhealthy eating patterns that include too much fast food, high refined sugar and fat intake, and yo-yo or crash dieting all put a tremendous strain on the adrenal glands as they struggle to maintain homeostasis in the body. Addictions to alcohol, drugs, and eating disorders will all cause your adrenals to work harder and increases the

risk they will become fatigued.

### #6: Pollutants and Chemicals (Addictions)
'Toxic load' is a phrase used to describe the overall level of toxicity in our environments. Air pollutants (from cars, industry), antibiotics in meat, pesticides on fruits and vegetables, even chlorine in our drinking water. All of these, and more, are chemicals that can have a material and negative impact on our overall health, including the adrenals. Some of these chemicals actually disrupt adrenal function, forcing the other parts of the HPA axis to adjust and fill the void.

## Four Levels of Adrenal Fatigue

All Adrenal Fatigue is not the same and symptoms can vary greatly between individuals. In a single individual the type and degree of symptoms can change over time. What I've learned, though, is that there are generally four different levels of Adrenal Fatigue, and these levels represent the development process of adrenal exhaustion.

### Level One: Initial Stress Response
This is the first phase of stress response, during which the body is still making enough of the hormones needed to adequately respond to a stress trigger. Blood tests administered while in this level would show higher levels of cortisol, adrenaline, norepinephrine, insulin and DHEA.

It's normal for us to slip in and out of level one several

times during our lives, and while sleep may begin to suffer, symptoms are rarely bothersome enough to report or seek treatment.

### *Level Two: Alarm*
Alarm bells start to ring as the endocrine system starts to divert resources from sex hormone production over to stress hormone production. In level two there is often a persistent feeling of being tired but hyper-alert: daytime alertness to function normally with a fatigue crash in the evening. Unhealthy dependence on caffeine or alcohol and other substances often develops in the alarm stage.

### *Level Three: Resistance*
The body demonstrates its brilliance in level two, adapting to prolonged stress by producing more stress hormones and fewer sex hormones. Testosterone and DHEA levels drop so that the endocrine system can keep producing more cortisol. Life and job function often still appear normal while in level three, but noticeable symptoms including decreased sex drive, regular infections and tiredness start to take their toll.

A person can hang around in 'resistance' territory for months, and sometimes even years.

### *Level Four: Burnout*
All the resources used to divert hormone production to cortisol production are used up, and even cortisol levels begin to drop. Low sex hormones, low stress hormones, and low neurotransmitters too. It's the crash that often arrives after long periods of significant stress. Here the symptoms can be noted throughout the body: extreme fatigue, apathy, depression, anxiety, weight loss, and depression, to name just a few. In burnout, you will

often find that you can't keep up with the day-to-day pace that has been "normal" in your life to this point. Recovery from burnout often requires a total lifestyle change, along with healthy doses of both patience and time.

# CHAPTER 3

## Overlooked, Misdiagnosed, Misunderstood

Adrenal Fatigue is somewhat controversial. The medical community is split as to whether there is a scientific basis for a diagnosis of Adrenal Fatigue, and many argue there may be other scientifically proven diagnoses to explain Adrenal Fatigue symptoms.

It's true there are a number of other illnesses that can be associated with Adrenal Fatigue: fibromyalgia, chronic fatigue syndrome, hypothyroidism, estrogen dominance, ovarian-adrenal-thyroid imbalance syndrome, and others. Generalized symptoms can often overlap. Proponents of Adrenal Fatigue believe that in some cases AFS is the underlying cause of these other conditions. Allow me to try to paint a clear picture of why I believe this medical conflict exists.

### Adrenal Insufficiency Versus Adrenal Fatigue

Adrenal insufficiency, known as Addison's Disease, shares many of the symptoms of Adrenal Fatigue, but they are much more severe. Addison's is often also accompanied by prolonged vomiting, severe muscle weakness, very low blood pressure or even shock, profound sleepiness or even coma. If you think this sounds serious, you're absolutely correct. A person with these symptoms may be in adrenal crisis and needs emergency medical treatment.

Adrenal insufficiency occurs when the adrenal glands are unable to function, if they're absent or have been removed. Most often adrenal insufficiency is the result of an autoimmune disease, where the body's own immune system attacks the cells of the adrenal glands. Infection, such as tuberculosis, can also be a cause. And in cases where the adrenal glands have been surgically removed there is obvious primary adrenal insufficiency.

Taking synthetic steroid medications like prednisolone, prednisone and dexamethasone can also result in adrenal insufficiency because it tricks the pituitary gland into thinking there is more than enough cortisol in the bloodstream, so it doesn't tell the adrenals to manufacture any more.

Endocrinologists warn that by taking adrenal supplements containing extracts of active adrenal hormone unnecessarily may render the adrenal glands useless and they may not work when they're needed most. Many serious illnesses, like rheumatic diseases, cancer, hepatitis C and more, share symptoms including fatigue, and self-medicating with these adrenal supplements may allow the underlying disease to progress undetected for too long before detection.

## History of Adrenal Fatigue

Once Dr. Thomas Addison first presented his theory on a

disease of the "suprarenal capsules" (today called adrenal glands) that presented as an anemia-like condition in the mid-1800s. Subsequently it became known as Addison's Disease. Addison's findings prompted further research and led to what became the field of endocrinology.

Later that century, physicians started using extracts from porcine adrenal cells (yup, pigs) to treat both Addison's Disease and the milder condition called hypoadrenia. "Adrenal Fatigue" as a term started emerging in the late 1990's. That's when Dr. James L. Wilson, a naturopath and chiropractor with three PhD's, started using it to describe a collection of symptoms that were similar across a number of tired, immune-compromised patients.

The debate between different factions of the medical community over the existence of Adrenal Fatigue has not changed much in the last century. What's at the core of this debate? The question of whether the line between health and illness is as solid as black and white, where a patient is either sick or healthy, or whether there is full spectrum on which there are many degrees between seriously ill and completely healthy.

## Illness-Wellness Continuum

In 1972, John W. Travis first proposed the concept of the "illness-wellness" continuum. Travis, founder of The Wellness Resource Centre in Mill Valley, California, opined that it should take significantly more than the simple absence of detectable 'illness' to determine whether someone was "well".

On the far left of Travis' continuum is early or pre-mature death. In the middle is a neutral point where there is no evidence of either illness or wellness. On the far right of the continuum is a high level of wellness. And in between the two points, from left to right, are:

- Disability
- Symptoms
- Signs
- Neutral *(no detectible illness or wellness)*
- Awareness
- Education
- Growth

This continuum, which by the way echoes the view of the World Health Organization, contradicts the methods of health professionals that only engage, diagnose and treat individuals when they are fully sick, on the left-hand side of the continuum: that is, exhibiting signs, symptoms and even disability related to disease.

Travis also believes that the "attitude" of each individual plays a significant role in where they fall on the continuum. Those with a positive outlook on life will have better health outcomes than those with a negative outlook on life, regardless of the presence or absence of laboratory-confirmed disease.

## Subclinical Versus Clinical

There are many illnesses that remain below the threshold of clinical laboratory detection: examples include rheumatoid arthritis, mild hypothyroidism and diabetes. Adrenal Fatigue is the subclinical syndrome of Adrenal Insufficiency, or Addison's disease. By the time the laboratory tests "prove" adrenal insufficiency, often the only treatment option is lifelong replacement of bio-identical corticosteroids.

Diagnostic procedures and laboratory tests are highly mechanized and do not take into account the significant uniqueness of each person's body. No detailed history, no look at nutrition, lifestyle or genetic factors through which to view lab test results.

Reliance on laboratory test results that are skewed to an all or nothing approach leave no room to consider Adrenal Fatigue Syndrome as subclinical to Addison's Disease, or that slight variations of results within a "normal" range may indeed be indicators of poor adrenal health in some patients. Doctors wearing these all or nothing blinders condemn patients like you and me to either suffer needlessly or search on our own for solutions.

Advances in preventive and so-called alternative medicine are helping those patients. In many cases they are able to stop disease development when it is still in this "sub-clinical" state so that it does not become more serious.

## Large Patient Pool

There is a growing swell of individuals like you who are willing and ready to take their health into their own hands and look for ways to help themselves to heal and feel better. According to Dr. Michael Lam (a Medical Doctor with a Masters of Public Health and certification from the American Board of Anti-Aging Medicine who specializes in Adrenal Fatigue and nutritional medicine), over 50 percent of the adult population will suffer from Adrenal Fatigue at some point in their lifetime.

At the time of this writing, 1.45 million search results were returned after entering "Adrenal Fatigue" into Google's search engine. That's a lot of interest and activity for a syndrome that traditional medicine doesn't readily recognize.

There is currently no simple laboratory test that can be identify or confirm a diagnosis of Adrenal Fatigue. This is, at least in part, what is at the root of the controversy, or conflict, between medical and health practitioners over Adrenal Fatigue (and other conditions).

In many patients, laboratory blood tests will turn up "normal", leaving the patient to feel like he or she is "crazy", imagining things, or a hypochondriac. Don't despair if this is happening, or has happened, to you! Keep reading. I can help.

## Medical Evolution

Let's remember that until very recently, the Western medicine community also failed to recognize chronic fatigue syndrome, fibromyalgia, chiropractors, naturopaths or Chinese medicine, which has been practiced for thousands of years. We only have to look back 100 years or so to find that "hysteria" was a catchall description for a host of "female" issues from fainting to anxiety, sleeplessness to irritability and nervousness, with questionable methods of treatment. Can it be such a stretch to think that medicine will catch up and Adrenal Fatigue will become a more widely recognized syndrome?

As more and more of us take our numerous physical complaints to our medical doctors, who tell us "your tests are all negative", and then continue to do our own research and take our health into our own hands, the medical community will have more and more reasons to adjust their approach.

# CHAPTER 4

## Adrenal Fatigue. Do You Have It?

As I just referenced in Chapter 3, other medical conditions can produce the same symptoms as Adrenal Fatigue. It is important to ensure you have identified, and been treated for, any other conditions or health factors that may be contributing to your symptoms before reaching a diagnosis of Adrenal Fatigue.

Adrenal Fatigue Syndrome presents with a combination of symptoms that together, along with the absence of any other formal medical diagnosis, brings you to the conclusion that your adrenal glands are under-functioning, or fatigued.

### Signs and Symptoms of Adrenal Fatigue

There are common signs and symptoms, experienced by nearly everyone with Adrenal Fatigue in varying degrees or intensity. These are:

- Fatigue
- Weight gain tendency, especially around the waist
- Frequent flu or other respiratory diseases or infections that last longer than normal
- Low sex drive

- Dizziness or lightheadedness when standing
- Poor memory and muddled thinking
- Low morning energy, as well as in the late afternoon
- Need caffeine or other stimulants to start the day
- Meals bring temporary relief
- Food cravings for fatty, salty and sugary foods
- Unexplained neck, upper or lower back pain
- Increased PMS, with periods that are heavy and stop, or almost stop, on about day 4, starting again on day 5 or 6
- Startle easily
- Feeling overwhelmed, trouble managing stress and responsibility
- Body temperature issues: cold hands and feet, warm face, hot flashes
- Unexplained hair loss, and
- Multiple allergies or sensitivities to food

## Physical Signs

### *Fatigue*
Fatigue is the biggest symptom of Adrenal Fatigue, and is present to some degree in every patient with AFS. In particular, upon waking in the morning, regardless of how long or how good a sleep you've had, feeling sluggish and just not able to "wake up" in the morning is a key symptom.

- Puffy, swollen eyes in the morning,

- Battling fatigue throughout the day, with a significant low in the late afternoon
- Disrupted sleep, and
- Feeling the most energetic in the evening

### *Weight Gain or Changes, Food Cravings*

- Abdominal fat accumulation that is unexplained
- Need for coffee or other stimulants to "get going" in the morning
- Cravings for fatty foods, and
- Cravings for salty or sweet foods

### *Blood Pressure*

- Consistent low blood pressure, and
- Dizziness when getting up from lying or sitting

### *Anxiety*

- Inability to relax, despite fatigue, feeling wired
- Feelings of low self-esteem and depression
- Panic attacks, and
- Feeling of adrenalin rushes

### *Hormones/Libido*

- Low thyroid function (hypothyroidism) that doesn't seem to respond to medication, and
- Low sex drive

### *Female Issues*

- Post partum fatigue and depression
- Recurrent miscarriages, especially during 1st trimester
- Painful menstrual cramps or unexplained missed periods
- Irregular menstrual cycle
- Ovarian cysts
- Uterine fibroids
- Endometriosis, and
- Premature menopause

### *Frequent Infections, Slow Healing*

*Examples include:*

- Recurring urinary tract infections (UTI)
- Unexplained eye infections, and/or
- Slower than normal healing of even minor cuts and bruises

## Mental or Emotional Signs

- Fuzzy thinking, brain fog or chronic racing thoughts
- Irritability, especially under stress
- Coping ability and emotions
- Can't focus or concentrate
- Feeling unable to cope with stress
- Mild depression, and

• Feeling frazzled or scatter-brained

**Miscellaneous Signs**

• Hair loss

• Temperature intolerance (sensitivity to heat and sunlight, cold hands and feet)

• Dry or prematurely aging skin

• Chronic tinnitus (ringing in the ear)

• Dark circles under the eyes that don't disappear with rest

• Body aches and joint pain, and

• Muscle weakness, loss of muscle mass

## Testing (or Lack There of)

Given the rift in the medical community over whether indeed Adrenal Fatigue exists, I advise you to take great care as you work to determine whether you indeed may suffer from the syndrome.

Consult your doctor, but be prepared for him or her to tell you nothing is wrong. Listen to your instinct. If you *KNOW* something is indeed wrong with you, be ready not to let your doctor's inability to help get you down.

So, visit your doctor, explain your symptoms, and ask for a general checkup and a comprehensive blood test to ensure you don't have other underlying nutrient deficiencies (such as low vitamin B12, iron or vitamin D, to name just a few), hormonal imbalances or other health conditions that need to be addressed.

If, after comprehensive tests have been completed, other causes have either been ruled out or addressed, and you still have the same symptoms, then you may consider the cause of your symptoms to be Adrenal Fatigue.

Unfortunately, your doctor or may not be willing to refer you to ***all*** of the recommended tests mentioned below because they are often not covered by insurance. If this is the case, you may also work with an alternative health care practitioner with experience in Adrenal Fatigue (if possible, as they may be hard to find). Discuss all your signs and symptoms with them, what other medical conditions have been identified and/or treated by your doctor, and ask for a saliva test.

Ask to see the actual lab results, and then use the information below to help you interpret the findings and balance that against what your doctor or practitioner is telling you.

### *Cortisol Tests*
Cortisol can be measured via urine, blood or saliva, and each doctor will have his or her preference. Many consider saliva the most accurate method, as it indicates cortisol levels at a cellular level.

A single cortisol test is not enough. Cortisol normally spikes in the morning, dropping off over the course of the day. So, in order to adequately determine the function of your adrenal glands in producing cortisol, measurements taken at a number of points during the day and mapped over a 24 hour period will tell your doctor much more than a single test.

If you are seeing a physician who doesn't have training or experience, or doesn't believe in Adrenal Fatigue, then the results are likely not going to be accurately interpreted. The laboratory's reference ranges are often so large that only the most extreme results – at either the high or low end – will be flagged.

What are those "normal" ranges? They will vary from laboratory to laboratory, and your doctor, if he/she is fairly progressive, may make adjustments to what he/she considers normal based on your health and other factors.

As a general guide morning cortisol of 5 – 23 micrograms per deciliter (mcg/dL) in the morning or between 3 – 16 mcg/dL in the afternoon would be considered "normal". The challenge is that even if results fall within this "normal" range, this may not actually rule out Adrenal Fatigue. It may be more helpful to look at "optimal" ranges, rather than "normal", or to take your results to an alternative medicine practitioner with expertise in Adrenal Fatigue.

### *ACTH*
Once your baseline cortisol levels have been mapped, an ACTH (adrenal corticotrophin hormone) challenge test may be useful.

You will be injected with an ACTH dose, which mimics stress in stimulating your adrenal hormone production. Your cortisol levels would be tested again. As long as there is a marked spike, showing as approximately doubled on your blood test as compared to the baseline cortisol test, your adrenals are likely functioning well. If the cortisol spike is less than double, it suggests under-performing adrenals.

## *Thyroid*

The thyroid also works on a feedback loop with the hypothalamus and pituitary glands, and this relationship is called the HPT axis. Remember that the adrenal glands are a part of the HPA axis, and optimal function is interrelated. They're all part of the endocrine system. Any weakening of the pituitary or hypothalamus glands, which occurs in Adrenal Fatigue, can result in lower thyroid function. The challenge is that the standard ranges for "normal" used by labs and the doctors who interpret the tests don't adequately consider the nuances of hypothyroidism, nor the fact that hypothyroidism itself may be caused by Adrenal Fatigue.

## *TSH*

The pituitary gland produces thyroid-stimulating hormone (TSH), which in turn prompts the thyroid to generate T3 and T4. If your thyroid gland is happily churning out adequate amounts of T3 and T4, your TSH levels will be lower because the thyroid doesn't need as much stimulation. On the other hand, if your T3 and T4 levels are lower, indicating you are hypothyroid, then your TSH will likely be higher, because your hypothalamus is sending more thyroid stimulating hormone, telling your thyroid it needs to produce more of the critical T3 and T4 hormones.

The laboratory reference ranges for "normal" TSH vary slightly lab to lab, but generally fall in the 0.4 – 4.0 units per milliliter range. Those suffering from Adrenal Fatigue often have poorly performing thyroid glands and the TSH level will be above 2.0. Perhaps not enough to prompt your medical doctor to order treatment, but, combined with other tests, may help you and your alternative medicine professional to reach a diagnosis of Adrenal Fatigue.

## *T3 and T4*

T4 is more abundant in the bloodstream, but T3 is actually responsible for most of the body's metabolic activity. Both T3 and T4 are comprised of free, or "unbound", hormones that are available for your tissues and cells to use right away, along with hormone that is "bound" to protein cells. The Free T3 and T4 is the most useful measurement as it gives a clearer picture to diagnosticians. For total T4, the normal range for adults is about 5 to 14 mcg/dL (micrograms per deciliter), while free T4's normal range is about 0.8 – 200 ng/dL (nanograms per deciliter). For total T3, look for results between about 80 and 200 ng/dL and 2.3 – 4.2 pg/dL (pictograms per deciliter) for free T3.

*Side Note: If you suspect you have a thyroid problem but the above thyroid tests are within "normal" lab ranges according to your doctor, consider having a full thyroid panel test completed, which includes TSH, Free T4, Free T3, Reverse T3, and Thyroid Antibodies. However, all of these tests are often NOT done by doctors as they may rely on TSH alone, which does not provide a full overview of thyroid function. You may choose to visit a progressive thyroid specialist or alternative healthcare practitioner instead. Iodine deficiency can also cause adrenal and thyroid symptoms.*

*If you suspect you have iodine deficiency, work with a professional to conduct testing and administer iodine supplementation (which is a delicate process that requires tailored guidance from a knowledgable, iodine-aware practitioner).*

### Blood Pressure Test

Comparing results of blood pressure tests between sitting and standing positions can reveal potential Adrenal Fatigue. The first reading should be taken after you've been resting for about 5 minutes and are fairly relaxed. Then stand up right away, and take your blood pressure again.

### Increased Pressure and Heart Rate

Your blood pressure should increase when you stand up in order to keep blood flowing to your brain. A ten to twenty point increase, along with increased heart rate, indicates healthy adrenal function.

### Static Rates Between Sitting and Standing

If you are very athletic, there may be very little change in blood pressure between the resting and standing positions. In this case, no change in pressure would indicate normal adrenal function.

### Drop in Blood Pressure

If your adrenals are unable to produce enough adrenaline and cortisol, when you take your second measurement upon standing you will notice a drop in blood pressure and you may feel dizzy.

### Saliva Test

Saliva tests are gaining credibility and recognition by medical doctors as reliable determinants of cortisol levels. Your doctor or alternative medical practitioner can order the saliva test, and this is the best solution.

Because your adrenal glands manage all of your stress responses, checking cortisol levels at varying times of the day are necessary to reveal fluctuations in the stress response that may be abnormal.

The test involves collecting saliva at four different points during the day (i.e. 8am, noon, 4pm and just before midnight) and then measuring the cortisol, estrogen, progesterone, DHEAS and testosterone levels.

## Self Diagnosing

If you aren't able to find a good healthcare practitioner to work with, or you simply can't afford one (some insurance plans do not adequately cover alternative health professionals or their referred testing), then here is some additional information to help you self-diagnose. Adrenal Fatigue is one of the few medical conditions that can be self-diagnosed and self treated. I did it, and I am feeling a whole lot better.

### *Home Saliva Tests*
There are a growing number of Internet sources for you to order your own saliva "home-test" to check your cortisol profile, and most of these laboratories are good and reliable. Just beware of websites that will also try to sell you vitamins, herbs or supplements. In other words, the bias will exist to try to show that you require the products they're selling.

### *Pupillary Response Test*

Physicians like Dr. Jeffrey Dach, Dr. Lawrence Wilson and Dr. James L. Wilson all talk about a pupillary response test you can do at home. This test can help reveal early stages of Adrenal Fatigue, but should not be taken in isolation as a number of other conditions can affect the results of this type of test. Pupillary response test is not as important in diagnosing Adrenal Fatigue as blood sugar control or blood pressure maintenance tests.

### *How to Do the Test*

You need a weak flashlight, or penlight, a dark room, a mirror, and a stopwatch (you can use an app on your smartphone).

*1.* Go into the dark room, and stay in the dark for a few minutes to let your eyes adjust to the dark.

*2.* Standing in front of the mirror, hold the light to the side of your head and shine the light from the side across one eye, not directly into it.

*3.* Keep the light shining steadily across the eye and watch your pupil. You should notice that it contracts immediately when the light hits it.

*4.* Time how long your pupil holds the contraction before it dilates, which it will... and then it will contract again.

### *What it Means*

The length of time your pupil holds the contraction before it dilates, and whether it "bounces" around dilating/contracting under the light, can be an indicator of Adrenal Fatigue.

The longer your pupil can maintain the contraction, the better. If your pupil can maintain contraction for 30 or more seconds before it dilates again, that's a great sign that you are not in early stages of Adrenal Fatigue.

Pulsing is also ok because it shows your body is adjusting. Where there are problems are when your pupil does not contract at all.

# CHAPTER 5

## Curing Adrenal Fatigue Naturally: Diet, Vitamins & Supplements

When you're under stress, your body needs more nutritious fuel than it would otherwise. The key here is ***nutritious***. Fast food just ain't it. Along with what you eat, when you eat is also important. Eating regularly – and eating enough – helps keep cortisol levels stable so the adrenal glands don't have to work quite so hard. The solution is to take in the right fuel and reduce potential dietary stressors to ensure our bodies run smoothly and optimally, which as a result, will aid in healing Adrenal Fatigue.

Based on my own personal healing experience with Adrenal Fatigue, plus many success stories of real people, I have endlessly researched the implications of diet in healing the human body – and the solution seems so simple. In curing Adrenal Fatigue, chose a diet that is simple, whole, and comes from nature; consisting of plant-based, high nutrient ***whole foods***. Eating a diet rich in plant-based foods is proven to decrease the overall risk of disease and places less stress on our adrenal glands, which I will address in more detail throughout this chapter.

Though this may not be renowned as a 'conventional' approach in a society full of marketing, fad diets and falsity, there are many educated, highly trained, and well-respected medical doctors who share this view (and from whom I have learned), who have successfully helped their patients become well again. You may also find other opposing methods out there that claim to cure Adrenal Fatigue, to which I disagree – I have tried these recommendations and found they made my symptoms worse and did not work *for me* in the long-term.

Dr. Neal Barnard has written extensively about preventing cancer with a plant-based diet. He references data that suggests the risk of dying from cancer increases between 14 and 50 percent for those who regularly eat red and processed meats and who consume high-fat dairy. Dr. Dean Ornish, Dr. John McDougall, Dr. Joel Fuhrman and Dr. Caldwell Esselstyn are also proactive nutrition experts, each promoting a diet that is plant-based and low in fat to prevent, or reverse, heart disease and other illnesses. If you do your own research, as I have, you will find other examples of medical doctors who have 'seen the light' and are promoting the power of choice in diet and lifestyle in reversing or preventing disease and dramatically improving how we feel. Adrenal Fatigue is one of the syndromes that can be reversed with a little education and effort, and it's my pleasure to help you along your journey.

## Diet

### Choose the Right Foods

#### *Plant-Based Foods*
A plant-based diet is centered on vegetables, fruits,

whole grains (preferably gluten free varieties for adrenal recovery), legumes, nuts and seeds, with little or no animal products. Some examples may include cucumbers, apples, leafy greens, broccoli, mushrooms, brown rice, berries, beans, lentils and peas, just to name a few. Colorful plant foods contain natural phytochemicals, fiber and antioxidants (which help protect our bodies from disease and supports our overall health), and provides our bodies with plentiful nutrients including iron and calcium. Though eating 100 percent plant-based is optimal, if you are transitioning, I do encourage you try to have at least 85 percent of your diet (the more the better) made up of these nutrient-dense, non-processed foods for faster healing. You will notice how much better you start to feel very quickly.

### *Whole Foods*
The opposite of processed. It simply means paying attention to eating food that looks as close to what it did while it was growing in nature, with the least amount of processing possible. Not that all processing is bad, either. The processing you do in your own kitchen, say making applesauce from organic apples, is fine and needn't be avoided. Ready-made foods or condiments that contain simple, natural, plant-based ingredients are also a fine addition to your whole food meals – you will learn to read labels like a pro.

### *The Carb Conundrum*
Carbohydrates are the macronutrient our bodies require in the largest quantities, as they are our main source of energy and fuel for our bodies (and our minds!) to function optimally – an essential key in combating low moods and energy levels in Adrenal Fatigue.

Many processed carbohydrate foods are considered 'simple carbs', which can metabolize fast and turn into quick bursts of energy highs and lows. Examples of processed simple carbs contain white table sugar, found in jams and jellies, soft drinks or candies, which contain little nutritional benefit. Avoid these processed carbs and opt for whole foods containing natural, simple sugars (like fruit), which are better metabolized by the body with its fiber, proteins, vitamins and minerals still in tact.

Many people fear fruit under the guise that it is the sole culprit for blood sugar spikes. This, however, is incorrect and depends how the sugars are harmonized with excess fats in the diet (particularly saturated fat), which I will address in the following section. During the initial stages of your recovery while your body is adjusting to its new diet, it's best to consume fruits and fresh juices earlier in the day, and as your Adrenal Fatigue stabilizes you may continue to incorporate more fruits into your diet to enjoy in abundance.

'Complex carbs' are also full of fiber, vitamins and minerals. They are satisfying as they take longer to digest, are utilized by the body for long-term energy release, and can actually speed up your metabolism so that your body burns calories more efficiently. Examples include whole plant foods like starchy vegetables (potatoes, sweet potatoes, yams, pumpkin and corn), and whole grains (preferably gluten free) – opt for brown rice over white rice, especially during the first phase of healing. These are all fantastic options to include in your diet at any time of day.

***Don't Avoid Carbs***

It's concerning to see so many men and women cut carbohydrates out of their diet in the hopes they will lose weight, when in reality, it can have quite the opposite result in the long-term. Avoiding carbs is a common mistake and can make Adrenal Fatigue worse, and here's why.

We've talked about the connection between hypothyroidism and Adrenal Fatigue. Carbs directly affect thyroid function. Carbohydrates get converted into the glucose (sugar), which works together with insulin to provide energy. Insulin is needed to convert T4 (the inactive hormone) into T3 (the active hormone). Low carbs = low insulin = low thyroid and increased symptoms, including long-term weight gain.

Cortisol, the main hormone produced by the adrenal glands, tends to increase when on a low carb diet because the body wants to balance out its glucose levels. This means it is a potential stressor to your adrenal system. If you're already suffering from Adrenal Fatigue Syndrome, or are susceptible and suspect you may have AFS, adding a low carb diet to a stressful job, poor sleep and maybe excessive exercise, and voila. You've just perfected the recipe for burnout!

Excess fat in the blood (particularly from animal products and processed oils) obstructs the delivery of glucose to our cells for energy, which overworks our adrenals, creates an adrenalin rush, and results in a blood sugar spike or insulin resistance. Some people like to treat this problem by eliminating carbohydrates from their diet. You could assume this *might* make sense, right? But this means most of their diet would be made up of fats and protein – and as we know by now, a whole host of health problems can manifest if the body is lacking an essential source of fuel to function properly.

Maintaining stable glucose levels will provide you with optimal fat burning efficiency, prolong your energy levels, have a positive effect on your mood and control your appetite whilst minimizing food cravings. So, don't be afraid of complex carbohydrates and natural sugars in plant-based whole foods.

### *Limit Gluten Grains and Concentrated Sugar*

These two culprits may contribute to impaired insulin response, HPA dysfunction and general inflammation. Lara Briden, a Canadian-trained Naturopathic Doctor now qualified and practicing in Australia, calls gluten grains and concentrated sugar "un-gentle carbs", and promotes avoidance for those with hormone imbalance issues like Adrenal Fatigue.

But Briden and other experts do recommend consumption of "gentle carbs", which are the carbs that do not promote inflammation. Root vegetables like beet, potato and sweet potato, and whole grains like brown rice, quinoa, buckwheat, millet or amaranth are great complex carbohydrates to feed an adrenal fatigued body. Eating moderate amounts is recommended as helpful in supporting adrenal function.

It is also very important to identify and eliminate any other foods that you are allergic or intolerant to. Food sensitivities are very common and may be worsening your symptoms. Common offenders include wheat, gluten, dairy, eggs, soy and many others.

## *What About Protein?*

Proteins are found in all foods (even in fruits and vegetables) in sufficient amounts for our bodies to thrive. For the initial treatment of Adrenal Fatigue though, it is recommended to regularly consume a small portion of protein rich food (plant-based, of course, like beans, nuts, seeds, or legumes) along with your gentle, slow carbs. This will result in even better blood sugar balance – effective for those of us with insulin sensitivities, which comes in hand with having Adrenal Fatigue. If you choose to consume soy products (fine in moderation if you are not intolerant or sensitive), opt for organic soy with the least processing possible, such as tempeh or organic tofu.

There are varying opinions regarding daily macronutrient ratios – what worked for me during my healing process was a measure of approximately 60% carbohydrates, 25% protein and 15% fat. Rather than being meticulous with this, I recommend that you simply ensure fat does not exceed approximately 20 to 25% of your daily intake, and make sure you are consuming more good carbohydrates than proteins to sustain sufficient energy levels. Everyone's protocol will be slightly different, as each person's metabolic rate and state of health is different. The overall emphasis is on whole foods, so you may experiment a little with ratios to feel what works best for your body and what will best enable you to stick to a whole foods diet. As your body adjusts to its new diet, begins to heal and balances its insulin, you may slowly increase your carbohydrate ratio to where you feel most satisfied.

***Facts About Fat***

Fats are an important part of our diet, but it is the quality and quantity of fat that we must be conscious of. We often hear about the benefits of a Mediterranean diet and like to attribute this to the usage of olive oil, but what is often overlooked is the general dietary pattern – a menu rich in unrefined plant foods with a very limited intake of dairy and meat.

What has worked effectively for many people who have suffered from Adrenal Fatigue is eliminating saturated fats (commonly found in animal products) and limiting processed oils, yet still enjoying the whole food version in moderation to receive full nutritional benefit (i.e. whole olives instead of olive oil, coconut meat instead of coconut oil, avocado over avocado oil, whole nuts and seeds over nut oils).

According to Dr. John McDougall, *"our bodies can synthesize most fats from carbohydrates and there are only a few unsaturated fats that our bodies can't make by themselves"*. As a result, there is no need to overload our bodies with excess fats and processed oils, which can overwork our pancreas and forces our adrenal glands to produce more adrenaline (which over time, can result in a multitude of health problems caused by poor diet, including Adrenal Fatigue).

Contrary to varying opinions, processed oils, including vegetable oils, olive or even coconut oil, are not healthful particularly for those suffering from Adrenal Fatigue. Hydrogenated oils, even if they sound like they come from a healthy source, like soybean, corn or canola, tend to be very inflammatory and can stimulate your adrenal glands – and when heated become rancid and carcinogenic. Oils are also calorie dense when considering their low nutrient value, as they are stripped of fiber, making them easily absorbed into the bloodstream – a recipe for easy fat storage.

Minimizing oils may be a challenge at first, so try cooking with vegetable broths, organic soy sauce (tamari), tomato juice or a dash of water when sautéing in a non-stick frying pan. In baking, you can replace oil with foods like applesauce or mashed bananas to add texture and moisture.

### *Calorie Restriction? Never.*
Unfortunately, our desire for immediate and fast results can often negatively affect our health. Crash diets and calorie restriction might get you to your goal weight 'faster' in the short-term, but ask yourself, will you be able to sustain the same dietary habits forever? Will you keep the weight off? And will this harm your health and your metabolism in the long-term? You *WILL* be able to get to a healthy weight and maintain it once you have healed your body and consistently eat healthfully. Patience and consistency is key.

It's really important not to under eat. Not eating enough or going long periods without a nutritious snack can put your body into more stress. It thinks there may be starvation on the horizon and goes into protection mode *(read: stress)*, putting more demands on your already-tired adrenals. Don't starve your cells of natural energy by avoiding or seriously restricting food – ensure to keep your body fuelled throughout the day and *NEVER* skip breakfast. This isn't a permit to stuff yourself, though –

simply honor your hunger and simply put down the fork when you are satisfied.

You will find that on a plant-based diet, you may need to eat quite a bit more in volume than you might be used to in order to get in sufficient calories for optimal adrenal function – this is because plant foods are packed with fiber and water, whereas processed foods are often contain concentrated 'empty calories' laden with processed oil and refined sugar. A wholesome bean salad may contain lesser calories than a small, greasy pastry, for example. Every individual's intake will be different, but try to aim for at least the same amount of calories that you were eating prior to switching to whole foods, or even more if you were restricting.

When you first start eliminating addictive, processed food out of your diet, you may find you still having cravings for them in the beginning. Whilst you are battling these cravings, don't be afraid to load up your plate with healthful plant foods, and snack often. The more satisfied you are, the less chances you will reach for that bag of chips!

### *Sweets and Treats*

If you find you're craving sweets, as many of us with Adrenal Fatigue do, opt for whole foods with natural sugars such as whole fruits. Instead of refined white sugar, you may replace with healthier sweeteners in moderation (minimize during the early stages of your healing process), such as coconut sugar, pure maple syrup, stevia, dates or pure date syrup. Avoid the use of artificial chemical sweeteners, which can wreak havoc on your health and metabolism.

Also beware that some cereals, breads, dressings and condiments can often contain white sugar, sometimes in surprisingly large amounts, so be sure to check labels and choose products with wholesome ingredients. Choose high quality bread made with whole grains (gluten free is best), instead of processed, white flour. Opt for gluten free natural oats, puffed brown rice or quinoa flakes, for example, topped with fresh fruits and seeds rather than highly processed cereals containing sugar.

### *Salt Surprise*
Healthy adrenal function requires sodium, and sodium is usually low in those suffering Adrenal Fatigue. Unless you are an individual with Adrenal Fatigue and high blood pressure, it's not a good idea to limit your salt intake. Be sure not to overdo it either – a pinch or two added to meals is adequate, and choose high quality sea salt. Celtic or Himalayan sea salt are great choices because they also contain other essential minerals and nutrients that the processing of traditional table salt has removed.

### *Ditch the Dairy*
Commercial dairy products are pasteurized, which makes the protein in the dairy product more difficult to digest. This leads to more inflammation in the body. How does the body respond to increased inflammation? The adrenal glands produce cortisol. Bingo. Avoiding dairy products helps reduce inflammation, which helps the adrenal glands hang on to its cortisol.

According to Dr. Michael Greger (physician and internationally recognized health and nutrition speaker), the consumption of dairy products has also been linked to various hormonal imbalances, acne, high cholesterol, cancer, heart disease and diabetes, just to name a few – yep, even diabetes. We are often misinformed that sugar (even from natural sources) is the cause of insulin problems, when in reality, an excess of saturated fat found in animal products (dairy, eggs and meat) creates excess acidity in the body, reducing its ability to regulate insulin levels. This is a bad news for anyone, particularly those of us with Adrenal Fatigue with already hindered insulin regulation. Why put your health at risk? Reduce your intake of animal products and make the simple switch over to organic milk alternatives, like almond, rice or coconut, if you're seeking a milk-type beverage.

### *Go Organic*

Many with Adrenal Fatigue Syndrome cannot tolerate the pesticides, herbicides, antibiotics or other chemicals sprayed onto or fed into our food as it is grown or produced. Eating organic produce wherever possible helps reduce our toxic load. Consuming organic ocean vegetables, like seaweed, helps to provide trace iodine, which supports thyroid function.

### *Stay Hydrated*

Fluid "dis-regulation" is a common problem in Adrenal Fatigue. The adrenalin released when the body is under stress increases the rate of urine flow, and according to Dr. Michael Lam, most Adrenal Fatigue sufferers are in some stage of fluid depletion or dehydration.

Make sure you are consuming enough spring or filtered water (a better option than tap water which may be chlorinated and fluoridated in many municipal water systems) to help your body maintain fluid balance. As a general guide, you should try to drink an ounce of water for each pound you weigh, per day (approximately 33ml per kilogram).

Additionally, consuming fresh coconut water (commonly referred to as "nature's Gatorade") also works effectively in hydrating and replenishing electrolytes.

### *Steer Clear of Stimulants*
Omit stimulants such as caffeine, cacao, energy drinks, drugs, and alcohol. The short-term boost you feel is detrimental to your recovery. They prompt your adrenals to make cortisol and adrenalin, mimicking the 'fight or flight' stress response, which is just adding to the burden on your tired adrenals. Try replacing cacao (or cocoa) with powdered carob if creating your own healthy treats. Carob makes a fantastic stimulant-free alternative for the faithful chocoholic.

Green tea is acceptable in moderation, which you may drink in replacement of your regular cup of coffee to help ditch the habit and cut caffeine cravings. It should be known that coffee is also a diuretic, meaning it eliminates water out of your body causing dehydration. Coffee is also acidic, and can be irritating to the stomach and upset digestion, and as a stimulant can keep you awake at night (to the detriment to your adrenals).

### *Teas Between Meals*
Another great way to hydrate and provide your body with nutrition, especially between meals, is to brew and drink caffeine free, whole leaf, organic herbal teas. Not black tea, due to its caffeine content, but teas with high antioxidant and anti-inflammatory qualities. Some

wonderful teas for adrenal support include licorice tea, hibiscus (flor de Jamaica), which is packed with antioxidants and vitamin C, and rooibos (or red tea), which has been studied to ease the symptoms of stress and lower stress hormone levels. Coldwater steeping may result in better concentrations of nutrients than hot steeping, particularly for hibiscus tea. Dandelion tea is also packed with vitamins and minerals, and dandelion 'coffee' is a fantastic replacement for those who are missing the rich taste of their regular coffee fix. Consume teas with caution if you are pregnant.

## Timing of Meals

Eating shortly after getting up is one of the most important changes you can make in addressing your Adrenal Fatigue. Overnight, your blood sugar levels drop, and the longer you wait in the morning to eat a nutritious breakfast, the bigger the demand you are placing on your adrenals to drive your body without food. Breakfast within 30 minutes of waking is ideal. If you can't stomach that, breakfast should be consumed within the hour.

An early lunch is also important, because your body will burn through its breakfast fairly quickly. The best time for lunch is between 11:30am and 12pm. Also aim for a solid snack between 2 and 3 pm to help you ride through the cortisol low that we know is coming between 3 and 4.

Aim for an evening meal between 5 and 6 pm, and plan for a high quality snack about 30-45 minutes before bed to help you weather sleep disturbances. (I will talk more about sleep in the next chapter.)

### *Snacking*

Those suffering from Adrenal Fatigue frequently have trouble maintaining blood sugar levels. Yes, your blood test results may show normal, but you may still exhibit signs of hypoglycemia: dizziness, anxiety, fatigue, and sometimes even a sense of being drowned. Healthy frequent snacking is one of the best ways to eliminate these symptoms. Get into the habit of carrying a snack with you wherever you go. Taking a nutritious snack just before bed might help you fall asleep easier, and stay asleep, because your blood sugar is in better balance. Here are some healthy Adrenal Fatigue snacking suggestions:

• Slightly salted snacks are helpful, as those with Adrenal Fatigue Syndrome are often in a salt depletion state because of the aldosterone dysregulation.

• Nuts – organic and raw tree nuts, like almonds, walnuts, cashews, pistachios, macadamias or pecans. Peanuts are not actually nuts, they're from the legume family, and in addition to being a common allergen they can also cause internal inflammation. Sorry peanut butter fans, no peanuts during the initial stages of your healing process.

• Organic and raw trail mix.

• Fresh fruits including apples, pears, berries, cherries, mango, stone fruit or bananas to sustain energy levels.

• Organic dried fruits, once your Adrenal Fatigue is stabilized, including goji berries, cranberries, blueberries, mulberries and goldenberries.

• Plain, unbuttered popcorn with sea salt.

• Hummus (made with organic tahini) and fresh vegetables like carrots, celery or bell peppers.

• Wholegrain crackers (could be made from brown rice, corn or quinoa) topped with avocado, tomato, radish, sea salt and pepper.

## Help Heal the Adrenals with These Foods

• Seaweeds (kelp, wakame, nori, kombu, dulse)

• Sprouts and leafy greens

• Whole food carbohydrates

• Whole fats in moderation, such as avocado and coconut

• Berries

• Carob

• Sea salt

• Miso, fermented naturally without MSG

• Red and orange vegetables

• Cruciferous vegetables, broccoli, cauliflower, kale

• Vegetable juices

• Ginger

• Almonds, chia seeds and flaxseeds

• Beans and legumes, when combined with wholegrain foods, and

• Licorice tea.

## Avoid Foods that Hurt Adrenals

- Coffee and black tea
- Refined sugars
- Alcohol
- Deep-fried anything
- Processed foods
- Saturated fats, including meat, cheese and eggs
- Addictive fast food and junk food
- Any food to which you are sensitive or allergic
- Milk and dairy products
- Products containing highly refined flours (pasta, bread, cookies, pies, cakes, etc)
- Gluten (limit where possible or eliminate if you are sensitive)
- Chocolate (containing cacao, cocoa, dairy or sugar)
- Rancid oils, nuts and seeds (even 'good' oils go bad, often quickly), and
- Artificial sweeteners, artificial ingredients.

## Supplements and Herbal Support

Common mistakes in Adrenal Fatigue recovery include using nutritional supplements and prescription medications improperly, often taking too much which can add extra strain on the body. Vitamin supplements and herbal medicines should only be used in concert with the recommendations in this book for a healthy, balanced diet, and never as a substitute for healthy eating.

It is also important to keep in mind that nutritional supplements are not regulated, and there are unethical producers out there who are more interested in sales volume and profits than your wellbeing. As well, lack of funding for studies into potential toxic consequences means there's little to no "standard dosage" information. And, how one person responds to one dose of a nutritional or herbal supplement can be quite different from another.

Okay, now let's take a look at some of the vitamins and herbs that have assisted many people in recovering from Adrenal Fatigue. You can obtain many of the vitamins and minerals mentioned from natural food sources, though some additional supplementation may help reinforce your healing process.

### Herbal Remedies

Herbal medicine is older than civilization. Animals of all kinds will deliberately eat specific plants as a way to address viruses, bacteria, worms or parasites. History tells us that Aboriginal and Chinese healers going back millennia have looked to the plants provided by Mother Nature to heal and keep the body in balance.

Here are some of the most common, and effective, herbs that are helpful in addressing Adrenal Fatigue.

### *Licorice Root*
### *(Glycyrrhizin Glabra and G. Uralensis)*

Licorice is widely used to treat Adrenal Insufficiency as well as ulcers. It helps influence the balance of cortisone and cortisol in the body. Adrenal benefits can be observed with just small doses of licorice, about 25 – 75 mg of standardized extract per day. Available in tablet or liquid extract form, licorice use is reported to have improved health benefits in the areas of blood sugar control, better absorption of iron, reduced inflammation, improved hormone balance in women, and healing of the lining of the gut. *(Note that licorice is not related to anise, star anise, or fennel, despite the flavor similarities. When looking for a licorice herbal supplement, be sure you are getting the real thing and not a product made with the less expensive anise.)*

### *Ginkgo Leaf (Ginkgo Biloba)*

It is commonly known that Ginkgo helps improve circulation, but it can also have a beneficial impact on stress levels. For thousands of years, the Chinese have also used Ginkgo for a number of issues from asthma and libido support to anti-aging. Ginkgo is also linked to beneficial brain function outcomes like increased alertness and memory, and reduced brain fog and mental fatigue. Ginkgo specifically helps with Adrenal Fatigue through its anti-oxidative properties, which help protect the adrenals from potential free radical damage.

Again, not all Ginkgo products are the same quality. Look for standardized extracts with 24 percent ginkgo flavones and glycosides, and 6 percent bilobalides and ginkgolides. Ginkgo is also available in liquid or tablet form.

### *Korean Ginseng Root (Panax Ginseng)*

Western herbal medicine practitioners use the main root of the Korean Ginseng plant to address physical or mental exhaustion. However, in traditional Chinese medicine it is used to promote longevity and reinforce vital energy. Recent studies have supported the use of Korean Ginseng root to assist with insulin sensitivity, better blood circulation in the brain, improved immune system and relief from some symptoms of menopause. If you have issues with sleep disturbances, it is not recommended that you take Panax Ginseng any later than midday.

### *Siberian Ginseng Root (Eleutherococus Senticosus)*

Sometimes called Eleuthero, this herb helps with mental processing, immune function and stress. What's actually happening is that the Siberian Ginseng Root acts like a mild stressor to the body, and it's the body's own response to the stress that accounts for the reported therapeutic benefits. For this reason, only those with mild Adrenal Fatigue should use this herb short term to avoid overwhelming the body's stress response system further and worsening the condition over time.

### *Ashwagandha (Withania Somnifera)*

This is an ancient Indian herb that has been widely used by India's Ayurvedic physicians for a number of therapeutic purposes, including improved function of the adrenal glands. Ashwagandha is a substance that helps the body return to normal. If cortisol is too high, taking Ashwagandha will help lower it. If cortisol is too low, Ashwagandha will help increase it. Taking Ashwagandha right before bedtime can help improve the quality of sleep for some people.

### *Ginger Root (Zingiber Officinale)*
Ginger root helps bring blood pressure and heart rate back into normal ranges, leads to increased energy and metabolic rate, which in turn helps to burn fat. It is also reported to stimulate digestive enzyme secretions that help the body absorb proteins and fatty acids.

Those with diabetes, liver disease or alcohol dependence should use caution using ginger root. Liquid preparations of ginger root often contain alcohol and/or sugar. In some preparations, ginger root also contains aristolochic acid, which may lead to kidney or urinary system disease. Signs include blood in the urine or an unusual change in the amount of urine produced. Pregnant or breast-feeding women should also avoid using ginger root products.

### *A Note About Stimulating Effects*
If you notice increased energy and less fatigue when taking any of the above herbal supplements, you may be tempted to celebrate. However, as pointed out by Dr. Michael Lam, the more pronounced you feel this stimulation, the more severe your Adrenal Fatigue, and you may actually be further depleting your adrenals as they work harder to sustain the stimulated state. If you experience noticeable stimulation or any other unusual side effect you should cut back and adjust your amounts.

## Vitamins and Minerals

There are a number of vitamin and mineral supplements that can help support adrenal function. Not all of these listed supplements will be appropriate or necessary for each individual, so you may choose to consume them through gentle food sources instead. The results of your saliva and other tests will help you and your health practitioner, if you have one, determine which of these supplements may be right for you.

### *Vitamin C*
Vitamin C is one of the key vitamins that can greatly assist recovery from Adrenal Fatigue. It's an antioxidant that works directly with the adrenals to produce cortisol. Vitamin C also enhances absorption of iron to help combat anemia. In addition, it's well known to help boost the immune system and protect against free radicals. 1000mcg is a good starting dose. Look for liposomal or buffered vitamin C.

*Food sources:* Raspberries, sprouts, papaya, kiwi, green leafy vegetables, tomatoes, hibiscus tea, citrus fruits, strawberries, amla (gooseberry) powder, citrus fruit, broccoli, red or yellow bell peppers.

### *B Vitamins*
B12, B6 and B5 all contribute to cell metabolic function. Taking high quality B supplements can help boost energy. Specifically, B12 helps with cell repair and red blood cell maintenance; B6 helps create adrenal hormones; B5 helps break down proteins, carbs and fat. Aim for baseline doses of 100 mcg of B12, 50mg of B6, and 1000mg of B5.

*Food sources:* Nutritional yeast, brewers yeast, nuts, miso, whole grains, potato, avocado, soybeans (and edamame), bananas, lentils.

## *Magnesium*

Studies suggest that as many as 75 percent of Americans are magnesium deficient, with produces symptoms of fatigue, depression, insomnia and muscle cramping. Too much magnesium can produce digestive problems, so start with a 400 mg dose to make sure you can tolerate it.

*Food sources:* Sesame seeds (or tahini), quinoa, pumpkin seeds, kidney beans, spinach, almonds, tempeh, green vegetables, wild rice, dates, flaxseed.

## *Selenium*

Selenium is an important trace mineral that is vital for healthy thyroid and adrenal function and also protects from cell damage. Ingesting too much selenium can be toxic, so if you choose to take a supplement, try no more than 200 mcg every couple of days, temporarily, during your healing process.

*Food sources:* Mustard, brown rice, brazil nuts, cabbage, chia seeds, arrowroot powder, mushrooms, onions, sunflower seeds.

## *Probiotics*

Probiotics help improve digestion, which helps the body process more of the nutrients in our food. They also provide immune system support. Look for a dairy free probiotic supplement that has at least 5 strains of bacteria, including Lactobacillus acidophilus DDS-1, and 10 billion CFUs (colony forming units).

*Food sources:* Sauerkraut, kimchi, kombucha tea, miso, pickles, olives, nut milks.

***Other Helpful Supplements***

These compounds may be helpful and are all easily available online and at most pharmacies or health food stores. Try Omega-3 (non-fish and plant-derived) to help reduce inflammation, CoQ10 to produce energy and maintain cellular function, Acetyl-L-Carnitine to boost metabolism, and a plant-derived Vitamin D supplement if you are not soaking up at least 15 minutes of sunlight each day.

# CHAPTER 6

## Curing Adrenal Fatigue Naturally: Sleep, Rest & Exercise

Sleep, rest and exercise all play key roles in managing and recovering from stress. Even exercise – commonly touted as a mandatory element in good health – can cause more stress if not done appropriately for your individual level of adrenal health. Falling through the cracks between sleep and exercise is rest. Simple rest. I believe that all three need to be given equal priority in your adrenal fatigue recovery plan.

### Sleep and Sleep Hygiene

How is your sleep? The importance of doing all you can to ensure you get adequate, restful and restorative sleep can't be overstated. Too many of us have let sleep take the backseat to other life priorities. We have developed bedtime habits that get in the way of proper and restful sleep. Whether the result is Adrenal Fatigue, or just perpetual exhaustion, paying attention to sleep hygiene can make a significant difference.

***What is Sleep Hygiene?***
Sleep hygiene is a term used to describe a number of practices that help ensure that nighttime is full of quality sleep, and daytime is full of alertness. The most

important of all the practices is to establish a regular, 7-day-per-week, sleep and wake pattern. Not a Monday-Friday pattern, and another for the weekends. This involves spending the right amount of time in bed. Here is a list of recommended and healthy sleep hygiene practices:

- Discipline yourself to reserve your bed for the two "s" activities, sex and sleep. Avoid watching TV, working on your laptop, or even reading.

- Eliminate caffeine, nicotine and alcohol. Alcohol may help you get to sleep, but as your body starts to metabolize the alcohol it wakes you up and disrupts your sleep.

- Exercise: vigorous exercise is okay in the morning or afternoon, *IF* this doesn't cause an adrenal crash, but restrict evening exercise to relaxing forms of activity like yoga (I'll get into exercise in more detail shortly).

- Make sure you get enough natural light. If you have been cooped up inside, whether due to winter or illness, find a way to expose yourself to some sunshine – the 'happy' vitamin. This also helps the body recognize the difference between day and night and reinforce the message that daytime is for waking and nighttime for sleep.

- No daytime napping. It can disrupt the important circadian rhythm of the sleep-wakeful cycles.

- Don't eat too close to bedtime, and remember that any changes in your diet may trigger sleep problems.

- Set up a bedtime routine that is relaxing. Avoid emotionally upsetting conversations just before you are going to sleep.

• Restrict the use of electronics in the half hour before bed and eliminate them in bed. The light from the bright screens works to trick your brain into thinking it is daytime. At the very least, put your screen on the dimmest possible setting if you must use the device in the evening hours leading to bedtime.

## Rest, Relax and Reduce Stress

Rest, rest and then rest some more. Once you've done that, find a good spot to sit or lie down, and rest. Okay, I jest. But just a little.

Examine the way you have been conducting your life, and notice how many times during a day you "push on through" because you think you have to "get things done". This is behavior that has contributed to your condition, and you must stop. Taking a 5-minute break between tasks is not going to make a significant dent in your productivity, but it is going to help you reclaim your health.

### Managing Stress

Stress is often viewed as something that happens "to" us, something that is beyond our control. With that perspective, we are victims, powerless to change how stress affects us. If this resonates with you, and sounds true for you, I have news.

You do have the power to choose your response to the external event. Mindfulness exercises can be very helpful in teaching how to separate the "judgments" we apply to nearly every situation, thought, action, and process in our lives from the things themselves. This helps to reduce the emotional responses, often stressful, and allows us to view things more objectively.

Worrying is an example. Decide to have a positive attitude and often a list of worries shrinks considerably. Ask yourself if the issue is something within your control, or outside your control? If it's something that is beyond your control, cross it off the list. Worrying is harming your health. If it really is a decision you must make, try making a note of it or write about it in a journal, and put it away for another time. But not just before bed, where it will interfere with your sleep.

Look for ways to shift your perspectives and attitudes on life, as necessary. Examples include practicing gratitude, appreciation, letting go, forgiveness, and exploring spirituality. All of these are powerful changes that produce positive change in how your body and brain experience – and perceive – stress.

## *Breathing – the Building Block of Successful Stress Management*

Most of the time we are unconscious about our breath. It happens automatically. One of the most effective things you can do as you start on the path to recovery from Adrenal Fatigue Syndrome is to practice deep, slow, smooth and rhythmic breathing, using the diaphragm. This helps release tension from the body, helps clear the mind, reduces fatigue and improves both mental and physical wellness.

### *Balance Your Life*
Too much work, too much doing things for others, and too little time to take care of yourself. That's a recipe that has to change in order for your recovery to have a shot at success.

### *Get Rid of Energy Suckers*
We've all known people who seem to suck energy out of the room whenever they're around. Got someone like that in your life? These people are energy-robbers, and you don't have enough energy to go 'round. Avoid them, even if only temporarily.

### *Happiness and Connections*
And did you know that happiness is a skill, rather than an attribute? Psychology professor and happiness researcher Sonja Lyubomirsky explains that only about 50 percent of a person's happiness is genetic. And of that 50, only 10 percent is attributable to health, income and looks. Still, there's a whole 50 percent that is a learned skill.

Research tells us that one of the strongest indicators of happiness and good health is the quality and strength of our human connections. Relationships and family, yes, but I'm talking about community connections too. If you read this and realize that you've been spending all your time caring for your kids and cleaning the house, or giving everything you've got to the office 12 hours a day, and you hardly spend any time actually connecting with people in your community, now is the time to start. What about your work connections? They can be beneficial, but if those are the only connections you've got in your life, it's worth taking another look. Take a class. Join a club. Check out a neighborhood fair or event. Find something that interests you, even a little, that your current schedule doesn't seem to permit.

Go ahead and create time for some romance, for some fun with friends and family, and leave the guilt trip locked in the basement.

Look for ways to spend quiet time with your self. Treat yourself to a bath, a walk, or a manicure, something that you enjoy, and then allow yourself to enjoy it!

### *Lighten Up With Laughter*
Laughter is one of the best activities for changing the way we feel.

Studies show that people who laugh regularly have lower levels of cortisol and epinephrine, lower blood pressure, and lower feelings of anxiety and stress. The studies also suggest that even faking laughter is beneficial: the body doesn't appear to be able to distinguish between the real thing and a manufactured laugh. No joking!

So, go ahead. Let yourself laugh, even if it is at your self.

## Exercise

It can be so confusing. On one hand, we know that we must get our heart rates up – cardio – in order to stave off heart disease. On the other hand, we know that exercise can precipitate an adrenal crash. We've been bombarded with messages about the importance of "working up a sweat", and we have been conditioned to think that if we haven't really "pushed ourselves to the limit", it wasn't really valuable exercise.

With Adrenal Fatigue Syndrome, you need to adjust all of that thinking. Exercise absolutely has an important role in recovery, but you have to create a strategy that is appropriate to the level of Adrenal Fatigue Syndrome you're suffering with. Doing the wrong kind of exercise, at the wrong intensity level, can trigger another crash rather than help you get better.

The trick is to design a strategy and approach that builds a personalized program that is suitable for your particular level of Adrenal Fatigue Syndrome.

### *Stop Intense Exercise*
That's right. Stop any intensive form of exercise for at least a month, longer if needed. Take a break from cardio and all other forms of strenuous exercise.

### *Restorative Exercise*
Many people with Adrenal Fatigue Syndrome will experience crashes triggered by regular stretching and strengthening exercise, which is often considered "mild" in the physical fitness world.

Adrenal restorative exercise is different, designed to help find balance and restore health by connecting the mind and body in a nurturing and restorative way. If your Adrenal Fatigue is in the early stages, level one or two, you may have success in restorative yoga classes.

For those with more advanced Adrenal Fatigue, even restorative yoga may be too much and trigger a crash.

### *Regular, Light Exercise*
As you start to heal, you will likely find you feel best with walking or light cycling. Do not overstress your body with strenuous activities.

You may find yourself totally drained after exercise, and as a result you've learned to avoid it altogether. Completely understandable, but except during an adrenal crash, it's not a good idea to totally forgo any form of exercise.

# CHAPTER 7

## The Road to Recovery

Adrenal Fatigue can take up to ten years or more to manifest, so it is important that you expect it to take some time to resolve, once you get on the right road to recovery.

Don't be discouraged if you don't lose weight immediately. You must remember that an Adrenal Fatigued body has endured a great deal of stress and must heal first. Your organs and hormones need to be working optimally in order for weight loss to occur. A slow release of weight will allow time for your body to rebuild and trust itself again and, as a result, you will keep the weight off in the long run. Be patient and kind to yourself, and allow weight loss to happen naturally.

You may feel tempted to rejoice and relax once you start feeling better, but keep going! Your new lifestyle habits are working. As time goes on, you can gradually reduce your dosage of nutritional supplements and maintain your newfound health through the power of lifestyle and diet.

### Recovery Process

Recovery speed and process is different for nearly every

person with AFS. Depending on the severity of your particular condition, other health implications, and your willingness to change, your process might take a few weeks, a few months, or even longer.

### *Preparation Phase*
This preparation period is critical for long-term success.

- 1 day to 6 weeks depending on the level of AFS
- May be no noticeable improvement in symptoms even though nutrients are changing for the better
- Reactions to nutrients may arise, resulting in feeling worse, adjustments need to be made
- Body is in process of healing and resetting internally.

### *Honeymoon Phase*
- A few days to 12 weeks or more depending on level of AFS
- Body handles stress better, reduced fatigue, anxiety noticeably diminishes, sleep improves
- Can be mini-crashes and setbacks, don't despair, recovery from these should be quicker than before you embarked on your recovery road
- Energy begins to return.

### *Plateau Phase*
It's virtually impossible to set a time frame for this period. It could be a few weeks or a few months. It could last for years and you could be completely symptom free, if you were in level one or two of AFS.

But the fact remains that the body must have time to rebuild itself, and for those in level three or four, the more advanced stages of AFS, this simply takes as much time as it takes.

It is possible that those of you with more severe AFS may need to slowly adapt to a lower level of overall energy function.

### *Expect Ongoing Cycles*
Recovery is not linear. Like recovery from addiction, major surgery, or any other major illness, the path of recovery is cyclical. Expect a spiral, and resist the disappointment or despair when you suddenly feel like you've suffered a setback.

I'll say it again: *cyclical mini crashes and recoveries are to be expected.*

The most dramatic and noticeable improvement will be in early stages of treatment. Then, after a period of time, you'll suddenly realize that the setbacks are becoming less severe, that they don't last as long, and over time, that the periods between these mini-crashes gets longer. You'll notice that your highs will be noticeably higher, your lows not as low.

Cycles, like a spiral, a little improvement, a little setback. Normal.

## Willingness to Change

All the best medical advice and support in the world will do absolutely no good if you don't follow the recommendations. If you continue with your poor diet habits, don't follow through on the exercise recommendations (either to exercise more, or less, depending on your level of AFS), and fail to take the suggested supplements, you will not see any improvement in your Adrenal Fatigue.

It also takes a willingness to pinpoint and eliminate the sources of stress in your life. This can be extremely difficult, sometimes requiring the termination of long-standing relationships, leaving a job, or changing your relationship with money.

Not everyone finds they are capable of making the choice - choosing their health and wellbeing over the status quo - but if you do, you will reap the rewards, feel better, have more energy and joy in your life. Speaking from personal experience, it is worth it.

Remember, you *DESERVE* to get well, and you *DESERVE* the time and energy to make it happen.

## Feeling Like Yourself Again

If you decide to walk down the road to recovery, and you take to heart the tips, suggestions and recommendations in this book, I know you will start to feel better.

You will have your libido back, your energy back, you may lose some excess weight, and you will once again have the energy and motivation to get through your day.

I have travelled this road myself, and have personally tried everything I suggest here and more. I have researched and tried much more than is captured in this book, and I have found what seems to work, what doesn't, and what is simply a waste of time.

I thank you for taking the time to read this book, and I wish you every success and good health.

# CHAPTER 8

## Bonus Adrenal Support Recipes

Please enjoy these plant-based, whole food recipes. They are among my favorites, and are now staples in my diet. These recipes, and others, have helped me recover from Adrenal Fatigue and are at least partly responsible for my ongoing good health.

### Smoothies and Tea

### Banana, Berry and Chia Smoothie

***Ingredients***

- ½ cup frozen wild blueberries
- ½ cup frozen strawberries
- ½ frozen banana
- 1 cup baby spinach
- 1 cup almond milk
- 1tsp. chia seeds

***Directions***

1. Add berries, banana, spinach and almond milk to blender and blend until smooth.

2. Pour into your favorite glass, top with chia seeds.

3. Makes 1 serving.

## Green Smoothie with Ground Flaxseeds

### *Ingredients*

- 2 cups fresh kale, spines removed
- 1 cup water or coconut water
- ½ cucumber
- 1/3 grapefruit
- 1 cup frozen pineapple
- 2T ground flaxseeds

### *Directions*

1. Add all ingredients to blender and process until smooth.

2. Pour into a glass and enjoy.

3. Makes 1 serving.


## Antioxidant-Rich Banana Mango Smoothie

### *Ingredients*

- 1 cup organic, unsweetened nut milk of choice
- 1 or 2 frozen bananas
- Pulp of 1 ripe mango
- 1 or 2 brazil nuts
- 1 tsp. Amla (Gooseberry) powder

### *Directions*

1. Add all ingredients into a high-speed blender.

2. Blend, drink, and enjoy.

3. Makes 1 serving.

## Refreshing Hibiscus Tea (Flor de Jamaica)

### *Ingredients*

- 8 cups water
- 4 bags of any organic zinger tea that lists hibiscus as the first ingredient OR use whole dried hibiscus petals
- Juice of one lemon or lime (OR blend in some raspberries)
- Liquid stevia to taste (optional)

### *Directions*

1. Add ingredients to a jug and refrigerate overnight, or for 8 hours minimum.

2. In the morning, remove the tea bags, or if using whole hibiscus, consider blending everything together.

3. Drink over ice throughout the day.

4. For a variation, toss in a few whole mint leaves as you blend.

## Whole Food Plant-based Meals

## Blueberry Buckwheat Pancakes (Gluten Free)

### *Ingredients*

*Pancakes:*

- 2 cups almond or other dairy-free milk
- 1 1/2 cups buckwheat flour

- 1 small ripe banana (or half a large one)
- 1 cup pitted dates
- 2 tsp. vanilla extract
- ½ tsp. Himalayan or Celtic sea salt

*Blueberry sauce:*

- 2 cups frozen organic blueberries
- ½ cup pitted dates (or ¼ cup date syrup or pure maple syrup)
- 1/3 cup water (more as needed)

### *Directions*

1. Whisk together dry ingredients in a large bowl.

2. In a high-speed blender or food processor, blend 1 cup of the milk, dates, banana and vanilla until it resembles a smooth paste.

3. Stir mixture into the dry ingredients, alternating with the remaining 1 cup of milk, until your batter is fairly thick.

4. Heat a non-stick skillet over medium heat (too high heat will result in under-cooked pancakes with over-cooked outsides).

5. Pour ¼ cup of batter per pancake. Cook until the pancakes start to firm on the upper side, then flip and cook until both sides are deep golden brown

6. Move cooked pancakes to a warm plate, covered with a towel, while you repeat the process until all batter is used.

7. While pancakes are cooking, prepare blueberry sauce. Place blueberries, dates and water into a medium-sized

saucepan and simmer.

8. Once dates are soft enough to blend and blueberries are no longer frozen, use a hand blender (or transfer into regular blender) and pulse until completely combined.

9. To serve, drizzle sauce onto pancakes and top with a handful of fresh or thawed blueberries and enjoy.

## Baked Breakfast Yams

### *Ingredients*

- 2 yams (sweet potatoes will do)
- 2 apples, diced and cored
- 2 small bananas, sliced
- Handful of raisins (optional)
- ½ tsp. ground cinnamon
- ¼ tsp. ground nutmeg

### *Directions*

1. Preheat oven to 350 degrees F.

2. Cover baking sheet with parchment paper, place the yam on the sheet and bake for 1 hour or until soft in the middle.

3. Transfer yams to serving bowls or small plates.

4. Slice open the yams, once lengthwise and twice across, then use fingers to squeeze the yam to bring the flesh to the top.

5. Add banana, raisins and apple pieces to the center, sprinkle with cinnamon and nutmeg.

6. Enjoy!

7. Makes 2 servings.

## Warm Quinoa, Roasted Pumpkin and Orange Salad

### *Ingredients*

- 1 cup quinoa
- 1 ½ cup vegetable stock plus ¼ cup reserved
- 2 large, juicy oranges
- 2 pounds pumpkin or butternut squash, cut into ½ inch cubes
- 1 cup chickpeas (cooked or canned)
- 5 shallot bulbs, sliced into quarters
- 2 cups rocket (arugula)
- ¼ cup raw walnuts
- 1 tsp. wholegrain mustard
- 1 tsp. organic tahini
- 1 T pure maple syrup
- 1/3 cup parsley, chopped

### *Directions*

1. Preheat over to 400 degrees F.

2. In a medium saucepan, bring quinoa, vegetable stock and juice of ½ orange to a boil (save other ½ for dressing later on). Reduce heat, cover and simmer until liquid is absorbed, 10 – 15 minutes

3. Peel other orange and cut into wedges.

4. Toss pumpkin pieces, chickpeas, shallots and orange pieces in a large bowl with 1/8 cup (or more, as needed) vegetable stock

5. Cover large oven tray with parchment paper and spread the pumpkin and chickpea mix onto the tray

6. Cook in oven for 20 – 25 minutes, turning and sprinkling with additional vegetable stock if needed, until lightly browned

7. Dry roast the walnuts in a non-stick skillet until browned, remove from heat and set aside.

8. Squeeze wedge of remaining ½ orange into a bowl and add mustard, tahini and maple syrup and whisk well until smooth.

9. Combine quinoa, roasted veggies and walnuts in a large bowl. Drizzle with dressing, add parsley, and season with sea salt and pepper to taste.

10. Serve on a bed of rocket and drizzle with extra dressing if desired.


### World's Best Vegan Chili

***Ingredients***

- 2 cup (heaping, go for it) sweet onion, diced
- 2 T. minced garlic, about 4 large cloves
- 2 jalapenos, seeded and diced
- 1 cup diced celery
- 1 large red bell pepper, seeded and diced

- 1 can (28 oz.) organic diced tomatoes
- 1 cup vegetable broth, with an extra ¼ - ½ cup reserved
- 6 T. tomato paste
- 1 can (15 oz.) kidney beans, drained and rinsed
- 1 can (15 oz.) pinto beans, drained and rinsed
- 2 T chili powder
- 2 tsp. ground cumin
- 1 tsp. dried oregano
- Sea salt to taste
- ¼ tsp. cayenne pepper to taste
- 1 tsp. hot-sauce (optional)
- Makes 4 servings.

*Toppings*

- Homemade vegan sour cream (recipe follows)
- Chopped green onions
- Fresh cilantro (coriander)

### Directions

1. Sauté onion and garlic with a bit of the reserve vegetable broth, in a large pot over medium heat, until soft and translucent (about 5 minutes). Season with a bit of sea salt. If they start to dry out, add a touch more vegetable broth.

2. Add jalapenos, celery, bell pepper and sauté until softened (another 5 – 7 minutes).

3. Add diced tomatoes (along with the juice from the

can), remaining vegetable broth, and tomato paste and stir, turning up the heat to medium-high.

4. Add drained and rinsed beans, chili powder, cumin, oregano, salt, cayenne and hot sauce. Bring to a slow boil, then reduce heat to medium-low and simmer until thickened (about 10 – 15 minutes), adjusting seasonings to taste.

5. Serve with homemade vegan sour cream, chopped green onion and cilantro.

## Homemade Vegan Sour Cream

### *Ingredients*

- 1 cup raw cashews, soaked
- ½ - ¾ cup water, as needed
- 2 tsp. fresh lemon juice
- 1 tsp. apple cider vinegar
- ¼ - ½ tsp. fine grain sea salt, to taste

### *Directions*

1. Put cashews in a bowl and cover with water. Soak for a minimum of 2 hours (8 hours or overnight is better).

2. Drain and rinse cashews, place in blender.

3. Add water, lemon, vinegar and salt. Blend on high until smooth, as long as 5 minutes. Stop to scrape the sides and/or add a touch more water as needed.

4. Once it is really smooth, transfer into small container and refrigerate. Cream will thicken as it sits.

5. Makes about ¾ cup.

## Sweet Potato, Lentil and Mushroom Shepherd's Pie

### *Ingredients*

- 4 – 6 large sweet potatoes
- 2 T Homemade Vegan Sour Cream (or to taste)
- ½ cup rice or almond milk
- 1 tsp. dried rosemary, or 1T fresh
- Sea salt to taste
- ¼ cup vegetable broth
- 1 large onion, chopped fine
- 2 garlic cloves, minced
- 6 oz. cremini or baby portabella mushrooms, sliced
- 2 cans (15 oz. ea.) lentils, drained
- 2 T red wine vinegar
- 1-2 T organic soy sauce (tamari)
- Sea salt, pepper, to taste
- 3T cornstarch or arrowroot
- 8 – 10 oz. baby spinach or arugula leaves
- 1 cup gluten free breadcrumbs (or you can use 2 cups crispy brown rice cereal pulsed in a food processor until it forms the texture of bread crumbs)

### *Directions*

1. Peel and dice the sweet potatoes. Put them in a large saucepan, cover with water. Bring to a slow boil, then lower heat and simmer until tender, 15 – 20 minutes. Drain and move them to a medium bowl.

2. Add the homemade vegan sour cream to the sweet potatoes, add the milk and mash until no lumps remain. Sprinkle with salt to taste, cover and set aside.

3. Preheat over to 400 degrees F.

4. While sweet potatoes cook, add vegetable broth and onion to a medium skillet and sauté over medium heat until soft and translucent. Add garlic and mushrooms and continue to cook, stirring occasionally, until the onions are golden.

5. Add lentils and their liquid and bring to a simmer. Stir in vinegar, soy sauce, rosemary, salt and pepper and cook on medium-low heat for 5 minutes.

6. Combine cornstarch with just enough water to dissolve and then stir it into the lentil mixture.

7. Add spinach/arugula, a little at a time, cooking until just wilted and still bright green. Remove from heat, adjust seasonings to taste.

8. Use a 2-quart round casserole dish, or two deep-dish pie plates, and evenly sprinkle the breadcrumbs over the bottom. Pour in lentil mixture, then spread sweet potatoes on top.

9. Bake for 30 to 35 minutes, until the potatoes turn slightly crusty. Remove from oven and let stand for 5 – 10 minutes.

10. Cut into wedges, and serve.

11. Makes 8 servings.

## Snacks and Treats

### Gluten-Free Banana and Walnut Muffins

#### *Ingredients*

- 1 ¼ cups organic almond flour (almond meal works too)
- ½ cup brown rice flour
- ¼ tsp. fine ground sea salt
- 2 tsp. aluminum-free baking powder
- 1 cup chopped walnuts
- 2 ripe bananas
- ¼ cup chia seeds
- 1 ¾ cups nut milk of choice
- 10 pitted dates
- ¼ cup sugar-free applesauce
- ½ tsp. vanilla extract
- 1 tsp. fresh squeezed lemon juice

#### *Directions*

1. Preheat over to 350 degrees F.

2. Put chia seeds and milk into a blender, set aside to soak for 5 – 7 minutes.

3. In large bowl, sift together flours, sea salt, baking powder and set aside.

4. Add applesauce, dates, vanilla, and lemon juice to chia/water and blend until smooth.

5. In another fairly large bowl, mash 1½ bananas with a fork. Chop the remaining ½ banana and set aside.

6. Add the blended chia mixture to the bowl with mashed banana and stir.

7. Fold in the flour mixture until just moistened. Do not over-fold.

8. Fold in ½ of the chopped walnuts and the left over chopped ½ banana.

9. Fill parchment-lined muffin tins with the batter, and sprinkle remaining chopped walnuts on top. Add a sprinkle of chia seeds if desired.

10. Bake for 20 – 25 minutes, or until a toothpick or knife comes away clean.

11. Makes 12 muffins.

## Vegan Strawberry Banana 'Nice' Cream

*(No ice cream maker required)*

### Ingredients

- 1 cup frozen strawberries
- 3 ripe frozen bananas (very ripe and frozen at least 24 hours)
- 2 T coconut milk (other nut milks work too but coconut is my fave for this)
- 2T shredded coconut
- 4 small fresh mint leaves

## Directions

1. Using the "S" or dough blade of your food processor, blend strawberries with the coconut milk until you've got texture like sorbet.

2. Add bananas and continue blending until well mixed, fluffy and creamy.

3. Serve immediately, or store in the freezer.

4. Sprinkle shredded coconut and add a mint sprig on top of each individual serving.

5. Makes 4 servings.


## Easy Date and Nut Energy Bars

### Ingredients

- 2 cups medjool dates, pitted and chopped into fine chunks
- ½ cup mixed chopped nuts (walnuts, pecans, almonds, macadamia)
- 3 T coconut flakes
- A palm full of chopped, dried fruit of choice (optional)

### Directions

1. Heat non-stick skillet over medium heat. Add coconut flakes, tossing or stirring consistently until golden brown. Watch carefully – the flakes go from brown to burnt in seconds.

2. Mash chopped dates in mixing bowl, then stir in nuts, dried fruit and coconut. If you prefer crumb-sized

pieces, you may pulse all ingredients in a food processor.

3. Pour mix into baking dish, lined with plastic wrap, pressing to about ¾ inch thick.

4. Refrigerate at least half an hour.

5. To remove from the dish, pull up on the plastic wrap.

6. Remove the wrap, and cut bars to desired size.

7. Can be re-wrapped and stored in the refrigerator and used as grab'n'go snack, quick breakfast, or dessert.

# A WORD FROM THE PUBLISHER

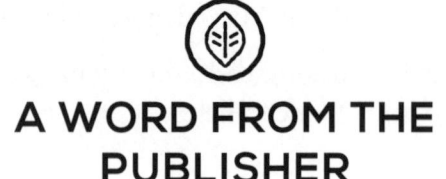

Hi, I'm Carmen, a holistic health geek with a passion for health, herbalism, natural remedies, as well as whole-food and plant-based lifestyles. After resolving various health issues I have struggled with for many years, I aim to inspire and help improve your health and longevity by sharing the tireless hours of research and valuable information I have discovered throughout my journey. Through the power of nutrition and lifestyle, with an evidence-based approach, I believe you can achieve your health and wellness goals.

***If you enjoyed this book, I would love to hear how it has benefited you and invite you to leave a short review on Amazon - your valuable feedback is always appreciated!***

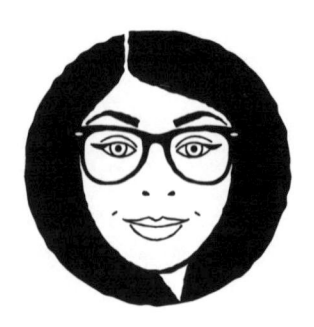

*You are invited to to join our **Free Book Club** mailing list. Sign up via our website to receive **special offers** and **free for a limited time** Health & Wellness eBooks!*

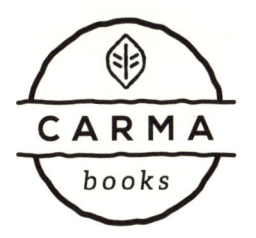

**CARMA**
books

'*A conscious approach to health & wellness*'

**carmabooks.com**

THANK YOU

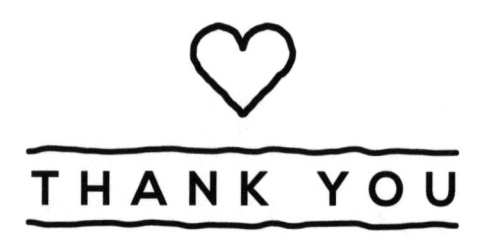

Printed in Great Britain
by Amazon